Parkinson's First Hero:
KING DAVID

Facing the Facts

C Randle Voyles MD

Copyright © 2012 Author Name

All rights reserved.

ISBN: 1530732301
ISBN-13: 9781530732302

DEDICATION

TO MY GREATEST FRIEND
MY CONFIDANT
MY IN-HOUSE EDITOR
MY LOVELY WIFE OF 44+ YEARS
ELIZABETH ANN

CONTENTS

	Foreword by King David	7
1	Making the Diagnosis in the King	9
	History's secrets hidden in full view	
2	The Psychological Response to a Diagnosis	19
	Redirection in life	
3	King David Seeks Help	25
	The neuroscience of Hope	
4	David Records His Legacy: Hubris in the Palace	29
	Creative dialogue of David, son Solomon, and Zadok the Priest	
5	2016 World Parkinson's Congress: King David interview	41
6	Epilogue by Zadok the Priest	51
7	About the Author	55

I am King David, son of Jesse.
I have Parkinson's disease.
To most in the world, I am the shepherd boy who slew Goliath;
That's right… with just a pebble and a sling.
Some know me as the King David who first united the kingdom of Israel.
I have Parkinson's disease.

Very few recognize the most important battle in my life.
Rest assured, it was recorded…* against my best wishes.
You see, my pride pushed me to battle in spite of my progressive malady.
I was almost killed by a Goliath descendent: Ishbi-Benob.
That changed everything…
I dare say, even world history.

I was recently noted to be the world's first person with Parkinson's.
I provided you ample clues 3000 years ago.
The clues were finally connected by a current scribe.**
He is a surgeon.
He also has Parkinson's disease.

*2nd Samuel 21:15 – 22.
**JMSMA. 2014; 55:14 – 1

C RANDLE VOYLES MD

Chapter 1

Making the Diagnosis in the King

History's secrets hidden in full view

David, the shepherd boy who slew Goliath, was first described in Jewish Scripture from 1000 BC. Later in life, David composed many songs, prayers, and praises that make up a large part of the book of Psalms in current Jewish Scripture and Christian Holy Bible. The Muslim world recognizes him as a prophet and the *Qur'an* has a named chapter attributed to David ("Zabur"). The story of David and Goliath is well known in the secular world and, indeed, is the title of a recent best seller[1]. Thus for the devout as well as the secular irreligious, King David, son of Jesse, has become a major character of the world's culture. Now, 3000 years later, it appears that he also may have been the world's first *described person* with Parkinson's disease. Furthermore, his most important battle *for world history* is little known.

Parkinson's disease is a common degenerative process related to a decrease of available dopamine (a neurotransmitter that "fires" nerve endings) in an area in the base of the brain called the substantia nigra. That specific area of the brain controls subconscious motor activity. In layman's terms, it is the control center that has taught you to walk and move your arms and fingers without thinking about it. The amount of dopamine slowly decreases and there are numerous backup systems; thus, the onset of symptoms is very gradual. Fortunately, or perhaps unfortunately, symptoms do not occur until there is about 80% diminution in the amount of dopamine production. The diagnosis is made most frequently at age 61-62. "Early onset" Parkinson's does occur as highlighted by the American movie star Michael J. Fox. The most clearly recognized presenting complaint is a unilateral tremor in a finger or hand. However, there are many other subtle non-specific symptoms - often recognized in retrospect – such as loss of smell (anosmia), slowness of movement (bradykinesia), and deterioration in hand-writing (micrographia). Later symptoms include the characteristic change of gait (shortened steps with shuffling and loss of free arm swing, usually unilaterally initially). While Parkinson's occurs in both sexes and all occupations, there is a preponderance in males (notably in type A personalities) and the neurodegenerative effects may be more readily recognized in individuals with occupations which require physical dexterity and stamina. Early on, the combination of symptoms can lead to **weakness and exhaustion** with moderately difficult tasks; later, there are major impediments with ordinary motor activities. When the effects of progressive motor disorder lead to a named diagnosis, the newly diagnosed member of Club Parkee (Parkinson's diagnosis) faces dilemmas: Do I tell? Do I keep on, not tell and hope no one notices? Should I take early retirement? Will retirement be forced on me? Very few have asked how this relates to King David....

Unique aspects of the history of David....

The Scriptures record more about the ages of events in the life of David than perhaps any other biblical character, certainly for the Christian Old Testament. We know that he encountered Goliath as a "shepherd boy" in his late teenage years. He became King of Judah at about age 30 and led his troops into many battles as the kingdom expanded. He reigned as King David for 40 years, seven years in Hebron and 33 years in Jerusalem. He ceased leading his troops into battle after a clearly recorded, life-threatening encounter at about age 61. David suffered from an unnamed progressively deteriorating condition prior to his death at around age 70-75. In his last days, he suffered from hypothermia and autonomic nervous dysfunction (both common in later stage Parkinson's). The throne was then passed to his son Solomon, who also served as king for the next 40 years.

When David used a pebble and a sling to kill the Philistine giant

Goliath, he made a place in history that persists to this day. *What is less well-known but more important* for the history of the world is his later encounter with another Philistine giant from the family of Goliath..... and his name was *Ishbi-Benob*. At that encounter on the battlefield, King David (now estimated to have been about 61 years old) was specifically reported in the Scripture as having become *weak and exhausted* in battle; he was about to be slain by the sword of Ishbi-Benob but was dutifully rescued by his trusted warrior named Abishai who killed Ishbi-Benob. At that juncture, David's men rendered a directive that was specifically recorded: *"You are not going out to battle with us again! Why risk snuffing out the light of Israel."*(NLT, New Living Translation) [2]

Methods and materials

A forensic investigative review of 3000 year old literature mandates a careful dissection of the recorded facts interspersed with some degree of creative thinking and extrapolation. To assign a modern day diagnosis to an individual from distant years might be called weird, nutty or whimsical ideation. After all, James Parkinson did not describe the *shaking palsy* until 1817. Thus, I plead not just for the reader's forbearance as I take a bit of liberty and editorial privilege but would ask that you read the following with the *trusting* assumption that the retro-active diagnosis of Parkinson's disease is correct. What are the clues from old literature that support a current diagnosis? More importantly, what difference does it make? Are there lessons to be learned by individuals with Parkinson's or with any unfavorable diagnosis?

The literature under investigation is called the Scripture (the recent TANAKH English translation) for Jewish friends and the Old Testament for Christians; both texts are quite similar for the period and writings of Kings David and Solomon. While there are dissenters about the authenticity of the Scripture, we will proceed under the assumption of literal interpretation of the historical material as God inspired. Again, we are detectives. The ancient recordings are backed by evidence of consistency from the Dead Sea Scrolls for at least 2300 years.

How good is your imagination?

Just suppose for the sake of argument that you are both a seer and sage in King David's entourage on a spring day in 940 BC. Your King is once again leading his men to battle against the Philistines. As long term counsel, you have a unique insight into the mindset of the aging Parkinsonian King David as he is the Alpha Male, Type A CEO of the Israeli forces. You had tried to provide wise counsel in personal matters earlier which he dismissed and suffered severe personal consequences. You recognize that his sense of self-worth makes it obligatory that he maintain his role as leader in the battlefield. He might ask: "Am I not the one God designated to slay Goliath? Surely, He wishes for me to slay Ishbi-Benob." However, the combination of bradykinesia, muscle stiffness and loss of agility – even in the face of dogged determination – sets the stage for the biblically-described *weakness and exhaustion* and failure in the battle field. David's men see it all; no doubt, they, just like you, have witnessed the King's deterioration. He has passed his prime! Is he a liability? You have a distinct premonition that somewhere someday there will be a reference to an emperor lacking clothes; does anyone dare tell him? But today, you, along with his supporting officers, face the uncomfortable task of relieving the highly respected king of his responsibilities on the battlefield – the very role that had made him unique in the history of the world. You try to console your dear King. (Club Parkee, what was the name of your Ishbi-Benob???)

More important for world history is what happened after the forced retirement for David. When he relinquished his role as military leader, he likely felt an initial emptiness with severe despair and some depression; paradoxically, he may have also been relieved. History suggests that he left his warrior role and wrote/collected much of what we know as the book of Psalms. He provided the father-mentor role for his son Solomon. David planned the building of the Temple in Jerusalem; he accumulated many of the materials. Solomon actually built the Temple and is credited with writing most of Proverbs, Ecclesiastes, and Song of Solomon (an alternate theory will be provided later). For the Christian world, David set the stage for and offered prophecy for the coming of the Christ child. Thus on review, David's early "retirement" from physical warfare was followed by literary contributions that helped shape the culture of most of the world. In spite of the neurodegenerative process that we now suspect to be Parkinson's disease, his major contribution came *after* his initial mandatory retirement from what he considered his major role in life. Club Parkee, take notice!

Introspection from a member of Club Parkee

Distinct clues from David's writings offer a glimpse into the life of one plagued by Parkinson's disease around 1000 B.C. These clues are more readily apparent to the attentive members of Club Parkee whose walk is both intensely introspective and, perhaps, a bit unstable. For example, one hindered by the gait disturbances of dopamine deficiency might anticipate that David would record: "He makes my *feet* like the *feet* of a deer and sets me securely on the heights... you widen a place beneath me for *my steps and my ankles do not give way.*"[3] Furthermore, David would proclaim "He *will not allow your foot to slip*; your Protector will not slumber."[4]

The psychological changes associated with a new diagnosis of Parkinson's are often more difficult to face than the initial physical impairment, especially if one is dethroned as a mighty warrior. David's initial effects of Parkinson's were certainly non-specific and prompted questions like: "What is wrong with me? Am I just getting old too fast? Am I over-reading my symptoms? Am I becoming demented?" The psychological load must have been particularly troublesome as the onset is insidious... yet progressive. With current radiological imaging (DAT scans and enhanced PET scans), the diagnosis of Parkinson's can be conclusive in many (but often it is not). A confirmed diagnosis is sometimes paradoxically a mixed relief. *My symptoms have a real explanation.* However, any initial relief is fairly quickly offset by the implications of Parkinson's: you have a progressive biochemical deterioration in the base of your brain (or worse); there is no cure; there are medicines that help with the symptoms but they have significant side effects; you will gradually lose physical control of mobility if you live long enough (but, so does everyone else!)

From despair and despondency to help and hope

New members of Club Parkee understand denial, despair, despondency, and depression! Even King David might find very little solace from his would-be comforters; "Yes, I know it is not cancer! You don't have to tell me that it could be worse! Yes, I know that there is meaningful life beyond a diagnosis! Yes, I am blessed with loving support! Yes, I know that God's love will prevail! But my days on the battlefield are over! Don't you know that self-pity is a rational choice???" On many occasions in his life, David recorded heart-wrenching despair with intense pleas to God:

1) "My God, My God, why have you forsaken me?"[5]
2) "How long will you forget me? Forever?... How long will I store up anxious concerns within me, agony in my mind every day?"[6]
3) "My days are like a lengthening shadow, and I wither away like grass."[7]

While self-pity and depression may have been rational responses for David, they were/are also counter-productive responses because a *depressive outlook hides help and steals hope!* ("I tried it once; it did not help!"[8]) Son Solomon recorded father David's admonition in the 12th chapter of Proverbs: "*Delayed hope makes the heart sick!*" David knew the enemies of despair and depression but they ultimately were overcome by help and hope. The great warrior realized that he was not the potter, but merely the clay. Interestingly, the historical Scripture records David's appeal for help from Yahweh and the subsequent transition to peace and solace... which led/lead to the challenges and recognition of a Higher Calling. *(The following italics are added to emphasize recognized deficiencies of the original member of Club Parkee.)*

1) "But in my *distress* I cried out to the Lord... He heard me from His sanctuary."[9]
2) "Keep me safe, O God, for I have come to you for refuge...Every good thing I have comes from You."[10]
3) "God, renew a *steadfast spirit* within me.."[11]
4) A recorded response from God: "Call on Me in a day of trouble; I will rescue you."[12]
5) David is consoled and records... "Your word is a *lamp for my feet and a light on my path.*"[13]
6) "I will bless the Lord who *guides* me; I know the Lord is with me... I will not be *shaken.*"[14]
7) "You delivered me from death, even my *feet from stumbling* to walk before God in the light of life."[15]
8) "I love the Lord because He heard my appeal... and rescued *my feet from stumbling* and my eyes from tears."[16]
9) "You have given me *hope* through Your Word... This is my comfort in my affliction!"[17]

10) With rejuvenated spirit, David asks to "be like the rain that falls on fresh cut grass, like spring showers that water the earth."[18]

11) "The LORD directs the steps of the godly. He delights in every detail of their lives. Though they stumble, they will never fall, for the Lord holds them by the hand."[19]

King David's Parkinson's disease in his old age

In the records of King David's last years, he had progressive disease typical for Parkinson's. He could not get warm – a condition referred to hypothermia. There is also a strong suggestion of genitourinary/autonomic dysfunction. Here is the record from the first chapter of the book of Kings (*King James Version*): "Now David was old and stricken in years; and they covered him with clothes, but he gat no heat. Wherefore his servants said unto him, Let there be sought for my lord the king a young virgin... let her lie in thy bosom, that my lord the king may get heat." A "fair damsel" named Abishag was brought to the king. She "cherished the king and ministered to him" but, the king *"knew her not"* (no intimacy; autonomic dysfunction).

Despite his old age, King David appeared to have been quite lucid and perceptive as implied in Psalms 41:5 – 8. "My enemies say nothing but evil about me. 'How soon will he die and be forgotten?' they ask. They visit me as if they were my friends but all the while they gather gossip and when they leave, they spread it everywhere. All who hate me whisper about me imagining the worst. '*He has some fatal disease*,' they say. 'He will never get out of that bed!'" Senior members of Club Parkee, does this sound familiar?

Now listen to this admonition which almost certainly describes King David. "Remember your Creator before *your legs start to tremble... before your shoulders stoop... before you become fearful of falling... before you drag along without energy along like a dying grasshopper.*" (paraphrased from Ecclesiastes 12:1-5, NLT). Again Club Parkee, how more descriptive could this be of Parkinson's disease 3000 years ago?

Some might ask why Scripture did not record a tremor in King David. First of all, he may not have had a tremor as 15 to 20% of Parkinson's patients never develop tremors. Secondly, he may have had a tremor that was not recorded per the King's insistence or reluctance of the scribes. After all, the king ruled with a "strong hand;" a tremor might have been regarded as sign of weakness, senility, or even demon possession.

Now let's review King David's features that are consistent with a diagnosis of Parkinson's disease... (Club Parkee, some of this is quite familiar).

> Age at onset: 61, typical for Parkinson's
>
> Gender: Male
>
> Psychological profile: Type A leader; compulsive
>
> Presenting symptoms: weak and exhausted with activity
>
> Response to early symptoms: denial, strongly implied
>
> Motor symptoms recognized by others: yes
>
> Impact on primary career: career ending
>
> Unilateral decision in retirement: enforced by others
>
> Expression of dismay and despair: clearly recorded
>
> Description of motor disorder: clearly recorded
>
> Progression from despair to hope: clearly recorded
>
> Improvement after improved attitude: clearly recorded
>
> Late symptoms: hypothermia and autonomic dysfunction

But the good news...

> Meaningful second career: clearly recorded
>
> Mechanism for improved outlook: Faith and Hope

Conclusion

History often hides its secrets in full view. Now 3000 years later, there is a high likelihood that King David suffered from a process like Parkinson's disease. While some may quibble with the retrospective diagnosis, they will have an even more difficult time disproving it. David's defeat of Goliath may have created the hero more familiar to most people today, but the battle that prompted his more important legacy – his written legacy – is the one with Ishbi-Benob. Clearly recorded. Nicely documented. *Secret disclosed.*

Members of Club Parkee, take heart. There are three messages:

1) Parkinson's disease (or a near equivalent) proved to be a catalyst for David's important written legacy.

2) His second career matured when despair and depression gave way to help and hope.

3) A positive attitude based on Hope and Faith is a powerful force in Parkinson's disease. Is faith a Glorified placebo effect? If so, what is the neuroscientific basis? Let's go to the next chapter.

The Lord is my shepherd, I shall not want.
He restoreth my (Parkinsonian) soul.[20]

[1] *David and Goliath* by Malcolm Gladwell (2013)
[2] 2nd Samuel 21:15-22
[3] 2nd Samuel 22: 34-37
[4] Psalms 121:3-4
[5] Psalms 22:1
[6] Psalms 13:1-2
[7] Psalms 102:11
[8] Personal commentary from surgical mentor Albert L. Meena, MD
[9] Psalms 18:6
[10] Psalms 16:1-2

[11] Psalms 51:10
[12] Psalms 50:15
[13] Psalms 119:105
[14] Psalms 16:8
[15] Psalms 56:13
[16] Psalms 116:1,8
[17] Psalms 119:49-50
[18] Psalms 72:6
[19] Psalms 37:23
[20] Psalms 23 (*King James Version* chosen for rich language).

Chapter 2

The Psychological Response to a Diagnosis

Redirection in life

"How would you expect me to feel? I am King David! I am a warrior king. I am the king who led my forces to unite the kingdom of Israel. Now those same men just banned me from the battlefield. Do you hear that? Banned from the battlefield! The battlefield is what made me! Excuse me, what did you just ask?.... Of course I know that I could not have gotten here without the blessings of Yahweh. And yes, I recognize that I suffer from an overly abundant sense of pride. It goes with the territory. But look where I am now. My men have taken away my sword. I feel like a defanged reptile. Could death have been much worse? Surely this is not the will of Yahweh. I am King David."

King David, the warrior king, most likely resisted forced retirement from the battlefield. Furthermore, one can also imagine that King David's first response to the earliest signs of his illness was denial. While the book of Samuel records David's life in great detail, much is left to the perceptive imagination of the reader. At the recognized risk of sounding egocentric, I have composed a short passage of how my symptoms progressed until my diagnosis was confirmed. With considerable hesitation and humility, I offer this as a weak proxy to an imagined response of King David. While every person with Parkinson's disease has his or her unique presentation with early waxing and waning of symptoms, the psychological responses likely share some common attributes.

A psychological case in point....

Something must be wrong! My first clue was a situational deterioration in my handwriting. Previously I took pride in my pretty handwriting that was generally very legible. What was bizarre about my deterioration is that it was stress related. For example, when I was multitasking at the end of the day, scurrying about discharging patients and preparing for my last operation, my handwriting was worse. Interestingly, I could take a deep breath and ignore (compartmentalize) the surrounding stress; my handwriting would revert to normal. When I returned to problem-solving, my handwriting again deteriorated. In retrospect, I was suffering from a dopamine brown-out as my relative level of dopamine had obviously decreased as a function of time and stress. *What's wrong with me? Am I just overly tired? Am I just getting older?*

One Saturday morning I was on call making rounds on our group of about 40 patients. My handwriting was particularly bad. I cornered one of my neurology colleagues who shared a common interest in trading markets. As an excuse to get his attention, I told him about my Goldman Sachs filtered trading method (a book in progress). Then I sheepishly asked him about my recognized inefficiency of handwriting; he promptly asked me about my sense of smell. I explained that my sense of smell had deteriorated for several years and I jokingly attributed it to a gift of God since I had to deal with so much foul-smelling pus and infections. That is when he alerted me to the possibility of early Parkinson's disease. "You don't look like you have Parkinson's," he said encouragingly but I sensed concern. "Why don't you come by my office?"

What would be the expected response from a surgeon to a suggestion that he might have Parkinson's disease? Of course, Google: What are the early symptoms of Parkinson's disease? Once "educated," I became hypersensitive to all aspects of motor function. My surgical skills did not seem to be affected but, on second thought, did I sense that I had to tell my hands what to do for ordinary tasks which I had previously done automatically at a subconscious level? Then a big question arose: *Am I a crock?* Next, I questioned the earliest form of foot drop? *It seems to be worse at the end of the day.* Was there an asymmetry of flexion between my right and left ankles? *No, I am a crock.* Meanwhile, my surgical practice continued to expand and it seemed that I was called upon to do more and more difficult operations with the pancreas and liver. I finished every day totally exhausted. Driving home after a long day, I reassured myself: *You are over 60 years of age. You should be tired. You don't have Parkinson's disease.* The days seemed to be become progressively longer; the night shorter (except when I was on call). I finally met with my neurologist formally. He told me that I did not have enough symptoms to make the clinical diagnosis (normal gait, no tremor, etc.). He suggested that we could just give it time or we could get a special brain scan called get a DAT scan (a nuclear medicine scan that can give images about the efficacy of dopamine transmission in the substantia nigra). I scheduled the scan and then canceled it as I thought I was over-reading my symptoms. *I am just a crock.*

Next, I questioned some asymmetry in my arm swing: my right arm seemed to swing less than my left. With Parkinson's disease, the initial symptoms are usually unilateral with the dominant side affected most often. I had told my wife of my concerns every step of the way. We took long walks. I knew that she would be supportive, no matter what. I alerted her about the arm swing and we both sensed some slight asymmetry. *Whoever taught you to swing your arms when you walk? Who says the swings have to be symmetrical? Are we both over-reading this?* In the ensuing weeks, I had a particularly heavy surgical schedule. At the end of one difficult day, one of my gastroenterology colleagues asked me if there were something wrong with my foot as I was not walking normal. I suggested that it was just because of my slip-on surgical shoes. However because of his unknowing prompt, I rescheduled the DAT scan -- after my surgery schedule on the next Friday. As you might imagine, the neuro-radiologist had already left the facility by the time the three-hour process was over. Educated by my study via the internet, I read my own scan. The results were unequivocal. What should have been a sharply demarcated area in the base of the brain was just a smudge. Diagnosis confirmed.

All the frazzled pieces of the puzzle fit together. The diagnosis was clear. *NOW WHAT? Tell? Don't tell? Just slow down and do minor cases?* Unfortunately the commitment of surgery does not lend itself to a part-time job. Even a simple operation can turn complex. There would be no way that I could take call and fulfill my responsibility to take care of the unexpected. Furthermore if I continued, I felt that I would have to inform the patient of my diagnosis. *I just have a touch of Parkinson's disease.* How reassuring does that sound? If I continued, wouldn't there be a time when I would put the patient's well-being at risk? Might that time be apparent only in retrospect? While I had avoided the courtroom in my surgical practice, I knew there was potentially a plaintiff lawyer who might rightfully ask me "Now Doctor, is it more likely than not that Parkinson's disease could compromise the safety of this operation?" It did not take me long to decide. There was little upside in trying to fight the battle as warrior-surgeon. The DAT scan was a blazing amber light – *no, it just turned red* – for my surgical career.

Common sense and medical advice was that I would function better in an environment with the lower levels of physical demand and emotional stress. After all, I had to adjust to a 75% reduction of dopamine in the control center of the base of my brain. Progression of symptoms would be real, expected, and inevitable. However the rate of progression would not be predictable. The best scientific studies suggested that delay in progression and preservation of function might be best achieved with aggressive exercise programs and good sleep; perhaps some various vitamin supplements might help. Next step: purchase elliptical bicycle and heart rate monitor. *Here is something I can do to help!*

Faced with an incurable process with a variable (likely prolonged) course, I had a forced re-look at earthly mortality and residual responsibilities. I had never planned for a medically-imposed retirement. How would I use my time? What am I going to do? *Honey, is lunch ready yet? I'm getting tired of watching Fox News.*

Just before my diagnosis was confirmed, one of my spiritual

confidants made the statement that retirement is an American phenomenon. He suggested that there was very little biblical material or instruction specifically about retirement. Only a few weeks later, my diagnosis was confirmed. One subsequent Sunday afternoon, I was riding my elliptical in the early days of retirement. I happened to be listening to the book of Samuel from the Scripture (audio via iPad).

"Once again the Philistines were at war with Israel. And when David and his men were in the battle, David became weak and exhausted... Ishbi-Benob was a descendent of the Giants... He had cornered David and was about to kill him. But Abishai son of Zeruiah came to David's rescue and killed the Philistine. Then David's men declared, "You are not going out to battle with us again! Why risk snuffing out the light of Israel?" *(2 Samuel 21: 15-17, NLT)*.

I stopped the elliptical and reread the passage. *Weak and exhausted*? A forced retirement? *Sounds all too familiar.* Did King David have something like Parkinson's disease? In chapter 22 David sang a song of deliverance: "In my distress I called upon the Lord... from his temple he heard my voice... I am saved from my enemies." He then made repeated references to motor impairment: "He makes me as surefooted as a deer, enabling me to stand on mountain heights." Do his metaphors have a real underpinning? Later, my search took me to the first chapter of Kings where I found even stronger suggestion of Parkinson's disease in David's latter days: hypothermia and autonomic dysfunction. *Why does everyone know about Goliath and no one appears to know anything about Ishbi-Benob?*

A Test for You: Extrapolation Skills

Scholars suggest that there was at least a 10 year interval between the time David was banned from the battlefield and his death. What did he do in his remaining years? Like many type A members of Club Parkee, he would not have just given up. Instead, he had to refocus his career – or perhaps his career was divinely refocused. Likely unknown to him at the time, he went on to leave his most lasting legacy: his writing. He collected and recorded the consoling scripture where Faith helped him overcome despair. Perhaps best known is the 23rd Psalms where he recorded *"He restoreth my soul."*

Now scratch your head with me. Was David not also at least partly responsible for collecting the Proverbs generally attributed to his favored son Solomon? (Read 4th chapter.) Did he not instruct Solomon to write an ongoing autobiography? (Read 4th chapter.) Did King Solomon revise and rewrite the last part of his autobiography after he had failed miserably as king of Israel? (Read next book in the series.) If so, think a little more deeply: would King Solomon have been better off if he had had Parkinson's disease like his father? Re-read the question. His legacy would have been much different.

Now, set your childhood story of Goliath aside and think with me. Had David died at the hands of Ishbi-Benob, how would history and much of the Scripture have been written? Take pause. Once again, has history hidden a secret in full view? Through literary forensics, is it possible to discover something new from 3000 year old material? Have the pages of history been shuffled by Parkinson's??? Is there not a distinct message for those struggling with a diagnosis of Parkinson's disease? Is this a message for me? Is Hope through Faith underestimated? Is there a more important mission than that of warrior surgeon?

Chapter 3

David Seeks Help

The neuroscience of Hope

King David had no oral supplement of dopamine. He had no oral dopamine agonist. He had no implantable deep brain stimulator. However, he sought spiritual Help which led to Hope; his subsequent written works have had a major influence on world history. How did this happen? What is the neuroscience of Hope?

The human brain is extremely complex. The behavior it generates usually seems rational, but not necessarily so. Some actions are generated reflexively at the subconscious level while others are a product of methodical conscious decisions. Whether decisions seem to be rational or irrational, they are all based on some form of chronic or recent conditioning. Our questions are the same as King David's: can we institute help and hope through mental conditioning to upgrade mood, attitude and outcome with Parkinson's disease? The answer seems to be an adamant yes. Is this a Faith gift of God? Again, seemingly yes. The mechanism is literally "in your head" as a function of neurobiology. Yes, an improvement is related to stimulating endorphins, opening up new neuro-pathways, and creating a *dopamine surge* in the important base of the brain.

How does attitude influence outcome? People make many decisions that seem to be irrational at a superficial level. For example, people purchase clothing, shoes and wine with the idea that the more expensive is better than the less expensive. Previous conditioning suggests that "you get what you pay for." Meanwhile, blinded wine tastings generally show a poor correlation between cost and tastes. As another example, people prefer red pills over white pills for pain medicine; another example of peculiar conditioning. Now, let's go closer to home for Club Parkee: in a recent blinded study (a study where patients don't know which treatment arm there are in) Parkinson's patients who were told that they were taking more expensive medicines had better outcomes than those with cheaper medicines; the medicines were the same. **Club Parkee #1: Mental conditioning influences mood/perception/outcomes.**

Not only does mental conditioning influence mood, but some seemingly insignificant physical activity may alter mood. In a recent study of normal volunteers, one half of the group was instructed to walk with an accentuated arm swing and long stride; the other half was instructed to walk with a diminished arm swing with short steps. (Does this sound Parkinsonian to you?) After that trial of a walk through the park, the group with the pronounced arm swing/long steps scored higher on a mood scale and made more optimistic choices. Thus manipulated behavior (that mirrors a Parkinson's walk) in normal volunteers negatively impacts moods and perception. Since most of us with Parkinson's disease have limited arm swing and shortened steps, it seems reasonable to extrapolate that our motor disorder may worsen a negative mood which further exacerbates the motor disorder. *So recognize the potential for the cycle: exercise with exaggerated big movements makes me feel better... really!* **Club Parkee #2: Physical conditioning influences mood/perception.**

In another study of healthy volunteers, one half of the group was instructed to go on a subway ride and freely engage in conversation with multiple strangers. The other group was asked to avoid eye contact and any conversations with strangers. At the end of the subway ride, both groups were tested. The group that engaged in conversation scored higher on mood tests and tended to make more optimistic choices; the reclusive group scored much lower. There is a lesson here for Parkinson's patients; we have a tendency to avoid the public and become somewhat reclusive. Accordingly, we have the following recommendation: **Club Parkee #3: Staying engaged influences mood/perception.**

The positive effects of hope through placebo are so profound that they confound randomized trials in science. Hopeful but blinded control groups (no medications; i.e., sugar pill) often derive measurable benefit just from being in a trial. This hope/placebo effect is even more pronounced in Parkinson's disease – estimated to be 25 to 40% of treated groups– because mental conditioning has a more profound impact on outcome with Parkinson's than in many other diseases. The differences are truly organic-derived as evidenced by dynamic MRI scans which confirm a dopamine surge in the basal ganglia in the hopeful non-medicated group. Can the hopeful placebo benefit be expanded for both new and old members of Club Parkee? For certain, complications from hope are few. **Club Parkee #4: Hope influences mood/perception.**

King David was not in a randomized trial. There were no medications for his motor disorder 3000 years ago. Nonetheless, one can readily discern that King David improved and went on to do his most important work after he relinquished his role as warrior-king. The organic pathway through which King David improved was mediated by Hope through Faith: "He restoreth my soul." To what extent can hope through Faith be applied to current members of Club Parkee? Does Faith improve as disease progresses? Does it diminish? Is Faith potentially available to all? Faith does not come in a pill but I would like more of it. **Club Parkee #5: Hope through Faith offers a powerful beneficial influence.**

> *Hope springs eternal in the humanbreast;*
> *Man never is, but always to be blessed:*
> *The soul, uneasy and confined from home,*
> *Rests and expatiates in a life to come.*
> *Alexander Pope, An Essay on Man*

The pathophysiology of Parkinson's disease is now better understood but the symptom progression remains quite variable. Patients who are late in the shuffled path of Parkinson's disease remember that – at least early on – they could consciously improve their walking, fine motor activity and even tremor... just by thinking about it. Later in the disease, it is more difficult to improve motor function by conscious effort. This leads to an important question: can one improve motor function on a more long-term basis with "chronic" positive mental stimulation? Data from several placebo studies suggest that the answer is yes, especially for bradykinesia. Tremors are less dopamine sensitive than bradykinesia; most tremors likely have a non-dopamine dependent mechanism. Rigidity is also less dopamine sensitve and likely is a function of chronicity. Thus it stands to reason that tremors and rigidity are also less effectively influenced by hope/placebo as the dopamine surge works at a different level. As disease advances, it is more difficult to improve bradykinesia with either the intrinsic dopamine surge or the oral dopamine supplements. In late disease the motor benefits of hope remain but to a lesser degree. **Club Parkee #6: Have reasonable expectations but never lose hope.**

In some studies, the benefit of placebos in clinical trials is short-lived; in some studies, it is chronic. Once the patients are told they are in the control group (no meds), the benefit usually disappears. In David's time, any improvement may have been called a gift of Providence through Faith. One might surmise that the benefit from faith might correlate with the degree of faith which is not measurable quantitatively. Furthermore, the level of faith may vary in the course of illness. Does faith get better or worse with progression of illness? There is obviously considerable variability, even within the course of one individual. However, the useful pathways still have an organic basis. The improvement, like the placebo effect, literally improves brain function. In later stages, motor function may deteriorate in spite of the hope/faith pathway. However, the person with faith may be more resilient and tolerant in later stages. What is the message for Parkinson's patients? What about their clinicians? **Club Parkee #7: There is no downside to Faith.**

***

Fiction often outlines truths more effectively than nonfiction. The next chapter is a creative writing of historical fiction. The <u>events</u> come from a literal interpretation of referenced scripture; the discussion is a product of fiction. In the structured dialogue between the elderly Parkinsonian King David, his heir-apparent teenage son Solomon and Zadok the Levite Priest, King David makes an initial attempt to enhance his written legacy as reflected in the book of 2nd Samuel. However, his pride is held in check by his son Solomon. We have no biblical reference but one can reasonably assume that Solomon became enraged when he learned about his prideful father's initial adulterous advances forced upon his mother Bathsheba. That's Bathsheba's story anyway... Let's turn the page...

Chapter 4

David Records His Legacy: Hubris in the Palace

A creative dialogue of David, son Solomon, and Zadok the Priest

"Zadok, write it *all* down!" said King David to the chief priest. "Write it all down from the beginning when I, as a shepherd boy, slew the giant Goliath with a mere sling and a pebble. Write down how I led our brave troops to many battles – how I conquered in all directions –how I ultimately united all the tribes of Israel. Without an accurate recording, our people may not remember how Yahweh led me to be your king."

"My King, it will be my honor to record it all," said Zadok. "Without question, you have led us to peace for the first time in history. You have provided safety in our promised land. Your borders extend from the Euphrates to Egypt. My King, this record – your written legacy - will be the most important chapter in history since the Torah of Moses."

Prince Solomon (son of King David by Bathsheba) held his tongue for as long as he could, then blurted out: "Listen to this donkey dung! One self-aggrandizing king selects a patronizing Levite priest to embellish his story. 'Accurate recording' you say? Then record how some of your very people call you a villain, a criminal, an adulterer, and yes, a murderer."

"Solomon, that's enough. You are excused" said the king.

"Vanity of vanities. All is vanity."[1] Solomon got up to leave the room, but abruptly turned and continued, "And on top of it all, you will likely record the great King David as 'a man after God's heart.'[2] What a great fairy tale. All is vanity. All is futile." He stormed out.

King David finally broke the extended silence. "Sorry for that outburst. The irreverence of youth. But... he is a brilliant young man. Blindly idealistic. Equally naïve. Loves to use big words. But Zadok, he does make a point and – I am sorry to say – he does have some justification for his disrespect. This Book of David must reflect the facts. It must include the bad as well as the good. "

"You are right, My King. If we don't include the unpleasant detail, someone someday will believe this to be a fairy tale."

"I will discuss our next steps with Solomon tomorrow morning. It may sound hard to believe just now, but we have been growing quite close. Every morning we work on a wonderful group of of verses about the verities – true lessons of life. We call them the *Proverbs*.

The next morning...
Solomon and Zadok were in the King's parlor. King David had not yet arrived. "Solomon" said Zadok, "the King told me about writing the Proverbs. Tell me how you two got started?"

"It's not a long story. I was just a boy when, one summer evening, he returned from another battle with the Philistine giants. He had no obvious physical injury but I had never seen him so upset. His armor bearer said that he had almost been killed by a Philistine warrior. The worst thing for him was that his soldiers took an oath then and there that he could never go to battle again."[3] Solomon paused, "I think he would have preferred to have died."

"Oh yes," said Zadok. "That was the battle with Goliath's grandson named Ishbi-Benob. One of David's men barely rescued him from that giant's sword. But how did that relate to Proverbs?"

Solomon said, "My father's despair only began to improve once he started putting to papyrus his feelings, his thoughts, his praises and prayers to Yahweh. Writing was real therapy for him. He called his collection the book of *Psalms*.

"Priest, I then encountered my own figurative Ishbi-Benob. You know, Zadok, everyone encounters some form of Ishi-Benob. I was 10 years old when I was introduced to the cruelty of life. To my dying days, I'll never forget that morning. My older half-brothers – Absalom and Adonijah – called out to me, 'Son of a whore, son of a whore. Good morning, son of a whore.' I didn't know what they were talking about. They kept taunting me. 'Son of a whore, son of a whore.' I bit my lip and tried to hide my emotions. I turned and ran straight to my mother Bathsheba. Dear Priest, she cried a mother's tears as she outlined a series of events that, frankly, sounded pre-rehearsed. She said she had no choice but to give in to my father's demands of lust. Of course, I wanted to believe my mother. Doesn't everyone want to trust their mother? Unfortunately, Absalom had already told me a different version. He claimed that my mother enticed the king by bathing completely naked on her roof. He said she set a trap for the king. He then said, 'Your mother is still hot.' Frankly, I want to believe my mother but I know her to be a manipulator who usually gets her way. So, I'm not sure to this day what happened. Still, every morning it remained the same: 'Son of a whore, son of a whore. Good morning, son of a whore.'

"I was so embarrassed that I stayed at home to avoid their taunting. I began to study even more intensely as a means of distraction. Who was I going to believe? Absalom or my mother? I had already concluded that my father was not innocent. As strange as it may seem, I then began to study Father's book of Psalms; I was impressed and, frankly, consoled by the praises to Yahweh. They seem to have been inspired by Yahweh. I followed my father's pattern and countered my despair with writing. I told my father and he was very eager to give me advice. Together we started the work that we now call *Proverbs*."

King David was making his feeble way into the parlor when he heard the word Proverbs. "Ah, the book of Proverbs," he said. "Yahweh and Proverbs keep father and son together." The king looked older than his years. Stooped. Short-strided steps. A shuffle. Very little facial expression. Even though he purposely carried a scroll in his right hand in an effort to mask his tremor, the infirmity – the shaking palsy of old age - prevailed.

"Zadok," said David in a dominating voice, "I am so proud of Solomon. He starts the first verses of the Proverbs with the profound statement that 'the beginning of wisdom is the fear of the Lord.'[4] I love that verse. I had previously recorded it in a collection of prayers and praises to Yahweh.[5] As you know by now, I call my collection the book of Psalms."

Solomon, showing a controlled agitation compared to the day before, said, "There you go again, Father. You love to say that all praise goes to Yahweh but now you heap praise on yourself claiming originality of the verse about the beginning of wisdom. Let's be clear. These Proverbs will be known as the Proverbs according to Solomon."

In an effort to avoid further disharmony, Zadok said, "Let's get on with our meeting. In the format that you two agreed on this morning, Solomon will introduce the topic of his choosing. You, my King, may offer some form of rebuttal, Solomon may respond, and I will be the impartial judge —with the final word as to what will be written. Solomon, what is the first topic?"

Solomon began. "Father, you are a gifted and successful leader. However, your pride overwhelms any sense of humility. You glow when you discuss victory but you dismiss the more important lessons of defeat. For example, the most important battle in your life was not the famed victory over Goliath but your loss to the giant Ishbi-Benob. Here's the lesson that you never learned: you lost because of a flaw of character. That flaw was too much pride – pride that forced you into battle when you knew you were not only too old but and you were not well. Pride led to your downfall. It should be recorded."

Zadok said, "King David, your response?"

"Shame on you for insulting and belittling your father," the King said. "And why was that the most important? Why would you draw attention to the near death of your father?"

"Father, if you will allow, it was that loss that led to your prolific writings. You even offered some belated mentorship for your children. For the first time, I got a glimpse of why some have called you 'a man after Yahweh's heart.' Thus you began to create your real legacy, which will be carried by your offspring and your writings. All of humanity will face their 'Ishbi-Benobs.' Your real story – portrayed with accuracy – will be more helpful to others. "

David asked Zadok, "What is your judgment on these issues? I have little interest in glamorizing defeat."

"My King, I think it is important to introduce Ishbi-Benob, but we can do it in a cursory fashion. The loss was real. Thus, we may attain the dual goals of providing accuracy and, perhaps, engendering an appropriate sense of humility for your readers. But, not to worry, young 'Ishbi' will be far overshadowed by the Goliath event. Rest assured that in a few years, no one will even remember Ishbi-Benob. Next, how to address your infirmity... I don't think it is necessary to record too much detail. We will state that you were 'weak and exhausted' by battle. You can provide clues to your walking disorder in your prayers to Yahweh in your Psalms. In addition, I have already recorded your prayer of thanksgiving where Yahweh 'makes your feet like the feet of a deer and sets you securely on high places,' [6] and how Yahweh 'enlarges the path beneath you so that your feet do not slip.'[7] An insightful reader will pick up on your shaking palsy someday."

"All right, but I have one mandate," said the king. "I don't want any references to the tremor in my hand. Someone may think that I am demon-possessed. My people know I rule with a strong firm hand. I will not allow any references to anything less."

"Solomon, is that acceptable to you?" asked Zadok.

"I will accept it. But recognize that you are patronizing the King at the expense of accuracy. His overriding pride still clouds his ability to remember the past. Pride that leads to downfall is really called hubris... Someone could write an accurate recording entitled *'Hubris in the Palace.'*"

"Solomon," said the disappointed King, "I taught you to honor and respect independent thinking. Now this is what I get: you think independently but your words fall short of honor."

***

"Solomon what is the next issue?" asked Zadok.

"Zadok, I have a concern that your goal is to 'deify' the so-called march to kingship," said Solomon. "In actuality, the march took a very devious – almost demonic - route. This man seemed to live for battle and he killed for sport. He was a most cunning schemer in his thirst for political control. He had no second thoughts about lying, cheating, or stealing to meet his goals. He proclaimed the Ten Commandments for his people but broke virtually all of them. His achievements may have been laudable but his methods were shameful."

"My King, would you like to respond?" asked Zadok.

"Zadok, my son seems to insist on criticizing his father. The insolence of youth!" began David. "I would hasten to remind him that one of the Ten Commandments is 'to honor your father and mother.' But, that being said, his portrayal has some truth in it. I did what was necessary. Someone may write someday that 'desperate times call for desperate measures'[8] and I lived in desperate times. My ultimate goal was to glorify Yahweh. The ends justify the means. Are we not sitting in my holy Jerusalem, my capital city?"

"And don't you refer to it as the 'City of David'? How does that glorify Yahweh?" asked Solomon.

"Solomon, you are interrupting your father," said Zadok.

"But Zadok," asked Solomon, "how did the king glorify Yahweh early in his life when he lived with the enemy – the Philistines? He actually was marching to war against his own kin – the Israelites- in the very battle where King Saul was killed on Mount Gilboa.[9] Some rumor that Father aided the enemy to clear his way to the throne. Others claim that he was there in the battle," said Solomon.

David shook his head. "Zadok, I have raised a disrespectful son. Solomon, I could have been there but I was not. I never lifted a hand against my people. Please note that Zadok has already recorded several times when Saul tried to kill me. I could have overcome him several times but I did not. I adhered to the law of Yahweh. I do not have his blood on my hands."

Zadok, sensing a need to redirect the conversation, said, "Let's clarify this issue by admitting the fact you, King David, lived with the enemy only because the enemy provided you a safe haven away from the vengeful Saul. I will record that you departed from the enemy troops before the battle began."

"Very well, Priest Zadok," said Solomon. "Ask the king with 'self-proclaimed' non-blooded hands to explain why he allowed the execution of Saul's seven male offspring by the Gibeonites. Was he not just protecting his claim to the throne?" asked Solomon.

David quickly said, "Solomon, the only way we could make atonement for Saul's massacre of the Gibeonites was to meet their demands to hand over Saul's offspring.[10] My forces had nothing to do with it. They had ample justification for their demands. King Saul massacred many and pillaged their entire tribe, I will add, without real reason. The blooded hands belong to Saul. I have no blood on my hands."

Zadok said "Thus it will be recorded."

"Zadok, you show extreme benevolence to your king - the king who alleges that there is no blood on his hands," said Solomon. "I ask for one question to offer final clarification. Zadok, I know you to be a good man. You have served Yahweh well. You are also in the presence of a powerful earthly king, King David, who has accomplished much and he is proud of it. As a final accomplishment, he had hoped to build a glorious temple to Yahweh. Zadok, would you ask the king why the prophet Nathan reported that Yahweh refused to allow David to build the temple?"

Zadok turned to David but said nothing.

The mighty king's troubled eyes stared in a fixed gaze – distant – as he peered into the dust of his past. Tremor worsened. More time passed. Finally he lifted his eyes and muttered softly, "Too much blood."

"I am sorry, dear Father. I don't believe Zadok could hear you."

"I said 'too much blood.' Yahweh said I could not build His Temple because I have too much blood on my hands." David sighed. "Now hear me clearly, Zadok," said David, redirecting his eyes to the priest, "It is advised that you record that I am planning and designing the temple. I am gathering materials. Say that the temple will be built by the next king. But, I insist, do not record that I can't build it because I have too much blood on my hands."

"How do you respond to that, Solomon?" asked Zadok.

"Zadok and King David can wordsmith their version of truth as their conscience directs," said Solomon. "But let it be clear that if I ever become king, I will always adhere to the truth and the Law of Yahweh. If I ever *chronicle* these events, my recording will reflect that King David was not allowed to build the temple because he had too much blood on his hands!"[12]

"Solomon, my beloved son," said the king, "you have grown up in a protected palace but this is a real world. Someday, you will be forced to make difficult choices. Odds are, you also will make an errant decision with consequences that will follow you every day for the rest of your life... also." He paused, in an effort to settle the tremor which was worsened by his agitation. "I hope that your 'enlightened' children will show more wisdom and sensitivity then than mine has shown today."

"Father, I will show wisdom," said Solomon. "I vow not to blindly pursue great riches or extend our borders. I will not gather a great harem like you did for my personal pleasure. All of the pursuit of worldly treasures is indeed *'chasing the wind'*. I will not try to extend the kingdom as *'the race is not to the swift... nor riches to men of understanding...but time and chance happen to them all!'*"[13]

"Zadok, Solomon has fallen back to the teacher mode," said David. "He has had the truly unique benefit of mentoring scholars from as far away as Egypt and Babylon. He often babbles about *'chasing the wind.'* Whenever he sees me making great plans for our palace, he proclaims *'Vanity of vanities... all is vanity.'* I have encouraged him to keep a diary as an autobiography. He has gone overboard, like he usually does, and calls this collection *'Ecclesiastes'* which literally means 'preacher' or 'teacher.' He continuously revives his work and I am certain that there will be many renditions in his lifetime."

"Father, I am surprised that you didn't bring up my book *Songs of Solomon*,'" the young man said.

"Zadok, I really don't understand why he would bring up such an embarrassing story," said David. "This work is outright bizarre. I don't know why he would record it and offer it for review. I hope it stays in the palace and never becomes public. His *Song of Solomon* describes intimacies of sensuality between two young lovers. There is not the most remote reference to the Yahweh. Really, I think he has spent too much time with the pomegranates. I simply don't understand."

***

Solomon continued with his questions.

"Father, you bring up the third broad topic that must be addressed in your so-called Book of David," said Solomon. "You must not mislead your reader with the idea that King David was glorious in all aspects of life. You succeeded in many battles but failed miserably in your family life."

"Be careful with this, Solomon," said the king.

"To start, the least painful part for me is the story of how your very son Absalom tried to kill you so that he could assume the throne.[14] My understanding is another of your offspring – Adonijah – is making a play for the throne as we speak."[15]

"Solomon, it seems that most of my offspring show more ambition than insight. Absalom and Adonjah thought I would skip over my older sons and give the crown to you."

"Father, forget your effort to dissuade me or change the subject. Your biggest personal failure is how you have approached marriage. Your first marriage was to Michal who just happened to be the daughter of King Saul. What a politically convenient arrangement! You left her for many years and only returned to 'retrieve' her after she was happily married to another man as if she were a piece of your property.[16] And don't forget wife Abigail. When you met her, she was married to a very wealthy man. The details are unclear, but the facts are that immediately thereafter, her husband died from a mysterious illness. Some rumor that he was murdered but the end result is that you took Abigail as wife and his possessions as yours."[17]

"Solomon, be careful with your accusations," said Zadok.

"No, Zadok, now *you* are interrupting me." Solomon turned back to his father. "The most hard-hearted story that ravages my very soul to this day is how you forced my mother into your bed. She was married to one of your leading generals. My mother told me she was forced to comply with your sexual advances. And then, you engineered her husband's death in battle so that you could continue your selfish desires.[18] Only for fear of her life does my mother live with such a ruthless man today. Mighty King, you are my Ishbi-Benob."

"Solomon," shouted King David. "I have had enough of this exercise. Your mother I love. No matter what she has told you, she repeatedly and intentionally approached me."

"How dare you talk that way to me about my mother! You saw her as a conquest – something to be conquered,' said Solomon. "Now you want to blame her!"

David took a long deep sigh. The room was silent, minus the rustling crescendo of the king's right handed tremor. "Solomon, let me strain to be calm. Hear me, son. Your mother knowingly and repeatedly put herself on full display bathing completely naked on her roof. She saw me on my roof top and she enjoyed my full gaze. I fell for her enticement."

David quickly turned to the priest in an effort to cut off the uncomfortable dialogue. "Zadok, I have had enough of this! However you must make a respectable record of these unfortunate events," he said in a stern tone.

Solomon, in an equally serious tone, said, "Father, your reconstructed memory shows how cruel and heartless you are. Your shuffling feet may have grown weak but your blind, self-serving ambition remains robust. Now let me also strain to be calm and respond to your earlier portrayal that my Song of Solomon is bizarre. I wrote the love story of a tender passionate relationship between two lovers because I knew you would never understand it. I knew you would never comprehend tender. You know only conquest. You don't know love!"

"Enough of this!" said David. "Zadok, you have the final word. Do you have anything more to say about my recorded legacy, the Book of David?"

"Nothing, my King, except that it will not be called the book of David as you have wished. No, it will be named after the old priest who first anointed King Saul and then you. It will be called the book of *Samuel*."

Ecclesiastes 1:1.
[2] 1 Samuel 13:14. "The Lord has sought for Himself a man after His own heart."
[3] 2 Samuel 21: 15-17
[4] Proverbs 1:7.
[5] Psalms 111:10.
[6] 2 Samuel 22:34
[7] 2 Samuel 22:37
[8] Attributed to Hippocrates around 400 BC
[9] 1 Samuel 28-31, especially 29:6-9.
[10] 2 Samuel 21: 1-9.
[11] 2 Samuel 7: 1-16 "I will raise up one of your descendants.....He is the one who will build a house – a temple – for my name."
[12] 1 Chronicles 22: 8. "And since you have shed so much blood in my sight, you will not be the one to build a Temple to honor my name."
[13] Ecclesiastes 9: 11.
[14] 2 Samuel 15-18.
[15] 1 Kings 1: 5.
[16] 2 Samuel 3: 13-16.
[17] 1 Samuel 25: 36-39
[18] 2 Samuel 11:14-17.

Chapter 5

King David Presentation

2016 World Parkinson's Congress

King David was interviewed at the 2016 World Parkinson's Congress in Portland, Oregon. That live interview has been recorded and can be reviewed by searching King David and Parkinson's on Google video or YouTube. (Click here if WIFI available https://youtu.be/KFXH9yijzmw.) If you lack Internet access, the following is a paraphrased transcript from the video.

Moderator on news channel with flashing *BREAKING NEWS*: "We are interrupting your regular scheduled program to bring you the breaking news from the World Parkinson's Congress in Portland, Oregon. Investigators have concluded that the world's first person with Parkinson's disease was none other than King David of Goliath fame. Equally remarkable, King David is taking questions now."

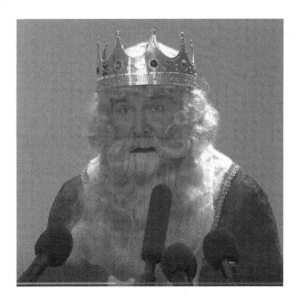

King David stands at a podium with his full regal dress, long gray hair and gray beard: "I am King David. 3000 years ago I left you many clues about my illness but it took a surgeon among you to make my diagnosis. (The King's tremor becomes exacerbated and he curses under his breath 'blasted tremor!') I have Parkinson's disease. I am happy to take questions."

News reporter from second row of audience: "Where did you report your typical symptoms?"

King David answers the question: "My specific symptoms were perhaps best described in the letter to my son Solomon. *'Remember your Creator before your legs start to tremble, before your shoulders stoop, before you become fearful of falling, before you drag along with no energy like a dying grasshopper'*" (Ecclesiastes 12:1 – 5, NLT).

Dr. James Parkinson (1783-1824), the English surgeon for Parkinson's disease is named, asked a question from the back of the room: "You describe precise symptoms. Where did you describe late stage disease?"

King David responds: "In later life, I experienced both hypothermia and autonomic dysfunction of Parkinson's as reported in the book of 1st King 1: 1-4 (paraphrased from NLT): "King David was now very old, and no matter how many blankets covered him, he could not keep warm [hypothermia]. So his advisers told him, 'Let us find a young virgin to stand before thee and cherish thee. Let her lie in thy bosom, that the king may get heat.' So they found a beautiful girl. She cherished the king. But the king knew her not" (i.e., no intimacy, autonomic dysfunction).

Mohammed Ali, the greatest boxer of all time, had a question proposed: "King David, you were also a great warrior like me. Can you tell me about the last battle that you lost?'

King David responds: "Tell the Champ I was once a warrior who could float like a butterfly and sting like a bee but I then became weak and exhausted with simple tasks. I tried to hide it but my men saw everything. My recorded loss has largely been ignored until recently.

Professional reader with images of King David (paraphrased 2nd Samuel 21: 15-17): *"Once again the Philistines were at war with Israel. David was in the thick of battle with his men. He became weak and exhausted. Ishbi-benob, a descendant of the giants, was about to kill David but his men came to his rescue. Then David's men declared, 'You are not going out to battle with us again.'"*

Moderator voice with pictures of Michael J Fox at various stages of his career: "Michael J Fox has noted your forced retirement with a particular interest. How did you respond to your forced retirement?"

King David's answer: "How did I respond? Like many here, my first response was denial, despair, and depression."

Professional voice reads several of King David's prayers in various Psalms: "My God, My God, why have you forsaken me? How long will you forget me? Forever?... How long will I store up anxious concerns within me, agony in my mind every day? I wither away like grass."

King David continues: "Despair made it all worse. God heard my prayers and my despair turned to hope. Listen! My motor disorder improved."

Professional voice reads several of David's Psalms of consolation: "In my distress I cried out to the Lord. You word is a lamp for my feet. You delivered my feet from stumbling. You make my feet like the feet of a deer; you widen a place beneath me for my steps and my ankles do not give way. Your Word is my comfort in my affliction."

Recently retired surgeon, now playwright and author C. Randle Voyles: "Well done, my King. You have been most helpful to so many. Any closing words for new patients?"

King David responds: "Of course. First, a positive attitude and a strong faith actually improve brain function in Parkinson's. Secondly, everyone here has untapped hidden potential. Find it! Exploit it! My early distress changed to hope. I was then inspired by God to write. Perhaps you have heard *'The Lord is my shepherd. He restored my Parkinsonian soul.'*

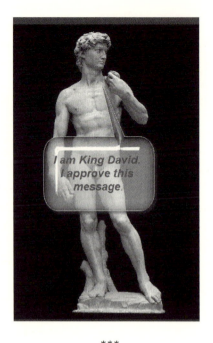

***

(YouTube ends here.)

Moderator: "King, we know you have a busy schedule but would you mind offering comments about the directives outlined by Club Parkee. They seem to be related to basic psychology. Would you have any comments?

"I am delighted to make additional comments about the seven rules which have been established by Club Parkee.

Club Parkee #1: Structured mental conditioning influences mood/perception.

To begin with, rule number one is no surprise. Sour attitudes lead to sour days; positive attitudes lead to better days. Man's behavior has not changed since the beginning of time. Solomon recorded this many years ago: *There is nothing new under the sun.*

"When Solomon and I began collecting the Proverbs, we envisioned a self-help book that would form the basis for helpful mental conditioning, a book that would last in perpetuity. We set lofty goals. Our Proverbs would lead to wise choices, successful living and bold leadership. You must understand that, at least at that time, Solomon was a youthful idealist but he was also naïve. He never forgave me for my initial adulterous relationship with his mother Bathsheba. I had hoped that the directions of the Proverbs would spare Solomon of some of the interpersonal problems that I had had in my earlier life. Unfortunately, during the course of his kingship, he showed the same weakness of man when imbued with too much power.

"Now, back to our lofty goals. The more we discussed the value of Proverbs, the less we valued our independent input as we were directed to our position and inspired by Yahweh. After several days' discussion, Solomon and I both concluded that the introduction to the Proverbs must begin by stating that the beginning of wisdom can only start with the respect, reverence, and fear of the Lord. In a similar fashion, my first suggestion to you as you embark on your road down the Parkee path: assess your Spiritual reference points.

"*The beginning of wisdom is the fear of the Lord*. We liked the verse. But, it was not original. A quick review of the Torah showed the introductory sentence of Genesis to be *In the beginning, God...* Take pause. Reflect a moment. Likewise, the first of the Ten Commandments states that *I am the Lord your God... You shall have no other gods before me*. In a later setting recorded in Deuteronomy, the call for wholehearted commitment of Israel was clear: *The Lord is our God, the Lord alone. Love the Lord your God with all your heart, your soul, and all your strength*. The same precise directive was given by Jesus in Matthew 22:37 along with the secondary directive *to love your neighbor as yourself*. Now many years later, the intrinsic law and governmental authority of most of Western civilization is based on that Judeo-Christian heritage. Such a heritage – a heritage that is established by centuries of conditioning – will also help your Parkinsonian pathway.

"Now back to implications for Club Parkee: The right mental conditioning will help direct your path. Your background mental conditioning develops from early childhood. I warned Solomon from early on. *My child, never forget things I have taught you. Store my commands in your heart. If you do this, you will live many years, and your life will be satisfying. Never let loyalty and kindness leave you. Tie them around your neck as a reminder. Write them deep within your heart.... Trust in the Lord with all your heart and lean not on your own understanding... Don't lose sight of common sense and discernment. Hang on to them, for they will refresh your soul* (Proverbs 3:1-5, 21).

"Yes, structured mental conditioning influences mood/perception and the beginning of conditioning, or you might say wisdom, is the fear of the Lord.

Club Parkee #2: Physical conditioning influences mood/perception.

"Excellent physical conditioning has a positive influence on your mood and perception, not to mention your physical health. Numerous scientific studies confirm the significant merit of aggressive exercise in Parkinson's disease. Thus I would suggest that you make no excuses. You will derive even more benefit if you find an enjoyable exercise which will generate an even greater endorphin stimulation and dopamine surge.

"By the way, there is abundant support for exercise from the Proverbs from 3000 years ago. *Wise words bring many benefits, and hard work brings rewards... Lazy people want much but get little, but those who work hard will prosper... A lazy person's way is blocked with briars, but the path of the upright is an open highway.* For many of you, exercise is a laborious task. My directive: just do it. Perhaps you will be amused by my analogy in Proverbs 14:4; *Without oxen a stable stays clean, but you need a strong ox for large harvest.*

Club Parkee #3: Staying engaged influences mood and perception.

"Club Parkee, don't become a hermit. Avoid being reclusive. Stay engaged because it helps your attitude. I recognize that you may want to avoid public exposure; I experienced the same sentiment during my last year, but I knew it was the wrong course. Besides, you should be reassured by this verse from Psalms: *I know the Lord is always with me. I will not be shaken, for he is right by my side.* Secondly, my responsibility as king was not lessened by my illness. I felt an intense obligation to continue the path that Yahweh set for me. Thus you will understand why it was important to record the following point regarding engagement responsibility: *I have not kept the good news of your justice hidden in my heart; I talked about your faithfulness and saving power. I told everyone in the great assembly of your unfailing love and faithfulness* (Psalms 40:10). Do you have unfulfilled responsibility?

"Club members, know that *kind words are like honey – sweet to the soul and healthy for the body* (Proverbs 16:24). Your responsibility to be kind did not go away when you got your diagnosis.

Club Parkee #4: Hope influences mood and perception.

"Modern neuroscience confirms the mechanism whereby hope leads to better outcomes. The concept is not new, but the technical confirmation by functional MRI scans is gratifying. The concept was recognized 3000 years ago. *A cheerful heart is good medicine, but a broken spirit saps a person's strength.* We knew that *Hope deferred makes the heart sick*. We also recorded that *a glad heart makes a happy face... For the despondent, every day brings trouble; for the happy heart, life is a continual feast.* I implore you to maintain hope for the human spirit can endure a sick body but who can bear a crushed spirit? (Proverbs 17:12, 13:12, 15:15; 18:14).

Club Parkee #5: Hope through Faith influences mood and perception.

"We have Hope through Faith because *Yahweh remembers us in our weakness. His faithful love endures forever. Since the Lord is my light and my salvation, why should I be afraid? The Lord is my fortress, protecting me from danger, so why should I tremble? 'Oh Lord I have so many problems but you are my glory, the one who holds my head high. Let your unfailing love surround me, Lord, my hope is only in you.' Yahweh frees me from all my fears. We who look to him for help will be radiant with joy; no shadow of shame will darken our faces. All humanity can find shelter in the shadow of Yahweh's wings. Thus I wait patiently for the Lord to help me knowing that he will hear my cry. Yahweh will lift me out of the pit of despair, out of the mud and mire. He will set my feet on solid ground and steady me as I walk along.* Club Parkee, *the Lord is merciful and compassionate, slow to anger and filled with unfailing love. Our trust is in his holy name* (consoling verses are from multiple sites in David's book of Psalms).

Club Parkee #6: Have reasonable expectations but never lose hope.

"Club Parkee, we all know that we face a progressive disease. As yet, there is no cure for earthly mortality, and in particular, for that associated with Parkinson's disease. However our prayer is that *Yahweh will show us the way of life granting us the pleasures of living with Yahweh forever. For now we are just moving shadows and all our busy rushing ends in nothing. Unless the Lord builds our house, the work of the builders is wasted. We put our hope in the Lord. When I am overwhelmed, Yahweh knows the way that I should turn.* That being said, *get all the advice and instruction you can so you will be wise the rest of your life. You should make plans but know that the Lord's purpose will prevail. Never lose hope* (various verses from Psalms and Proverbs).

Club Parkee #7: There is no downside to Faith.

"Many in the audience may be dissuaded by strong references to Faith. That is an unfortunate consequence of your current era in time. However, there is once again *nothing new under the sun* as world history has frequently been witness to errant culture. There is a reason that I started the very first verse of Psalms for this purpose: *There is joy in those who do not join in with mockers but rather delight in the law of the Lord, meditating on it day and night. Only fools say there is no God. Day by day, the Lord takes care of the innocent, and they will receive an inheritance that lasts forever. Accordingly, my prayer to Yahweh is to test me and know my anxious thoughts, but point out anything in me that offends you and lead me along the path of everlasting life.*

***

"Club Parkee, in conclusion, I am King David. I am best known to many of you because of my battle with Goliath. Now you understand that the more important battle was the one with Ishbi-Benob and it only came about because I was blessed with Parkinson's disease. I have shuffled down the same path that you are on. I know despair and despondency and yes regrettably depression that you may be facing. I sought help and found peace. You are not alone. The Good Shepherd will hold your hand."

[King David then turned from the podium and shuffled to a seat in the center of the stage. The room was absolutely silent as he took his seat and lifted the beautiful, ancient lyre. The lights in the room grew dim with the exception of the spotlight on the King. He began to play. Soft music. Peaceful. Soothing. He lifted his head and began to quote the 23rd Psalm as only King David could do.]

The Lord is my shepherd; I shall not want.
He makes me to lie down in green pastures;
He leads me beside the still waters.
He restoreth my soul;
He leads me in the paths of righteousness for his namesake.
Yea, though I walk through the valley of the shadow of death,
I will fear no evil;

For you are with me; your rod and your staff, they comfort me.
You prepare a table before me in the presence of mine enemies;
You anoint my head with oil; my cup runs over.
Surely goodness and mercy shall follow me all the days of my life.
And I will dwell in the house of the Lord forever...

...forever...

CHAPTER 6

Epilogue by Zadok the Priest

I am the Levite priest named Zadok. I served both King David and King Solomon. My most important historical contribution was the anointing of King Solomon about 3000 years ago. You Brits may know me more for the coronation anthem that was titled in my name and written by George Frederick Handel; *Zadok the Priest* has been sung at every anointing of the British sovereign since King George II in 1727. The lyrics are actually taken from the biblical account of the anointing of King Solomon; the words of the song ("God save the King!") have been used since the English coronation of King Edgar in 973.

Back to the subject at hand... I trust you now have a better understanding of the importance of the world's first recognized biography. King David was and has been a mighty influence in the history of the world. The described conflict and efforts toward resolution provide the templates for many/most/all subsequent literary works as well as current geopolitical conflict. Can you recall how many times leaders have made ambitious decisions supported by self-declared Providential guidance? The ambitions of errant humanity – whether described by Shakespeare, directed by Machiavelli, or recorded in the annals of history - share roots from 3000 years ago. Also, note the initial battles between David and the Philistines are ongoing as Palestinians (same word derivation is Philistine) continue to inhabit the coastal strip of land known as the Gaza Strip.

Most recently, King David seemed pleased that he has finally been recognized – 3000 years later - as being the first person in the world with a diagnosis of Parkinson's disease. Now he has an explanation for the muscle stiffness and exhaustion that led to his defeat by Ishbi-Benob. He was surprised that it took so long for your so-called scientists to make a diagnosis, relating that he gave them bountiful clues of his motor disorders in the Book of Samuel and Psalms. He is also keen to report to YOU, the reader, that once he perceived that he was not well - that he was a mere earthly mortal - he then recognized the importance of making every day as meaningful as possible. He was even bold enough to say that had it not been for his infirmity of the shaking palsy, his greatest works – his real legacy – would never been recorded. So, members of Club Parkee, perk up!

However, you don't have to have Parkinson's disease to appreciate the praises and consolation of the Psalms as well as the good directions of Proverbs. There is no end to the figurative "Ishbi-Benobs" that people have encountered over the centuries. Hopefully, you can lean on the Love of Yahweh in times of trouble and experience renewed agility with feet "like the feet of deer."

Perhaps, David's display of "Hubris in the Palace" may have explained some of the mystery of the books of the Bible. Ecclesiastes and Song of Solomon may make more sense to you. Make sure you read the next book in the series for more information. Solomon's failure as king is being addressed in a separate book entitled *Parkinson's First Son: King Solomon;* however, *Good Sex, Great Songs, and Old Jews* could be a quirky, perhaps more descriptive subtitle. Also, you detail-oriented biblical historians, note the obvious differences in the books of Samuel and Chronicles in the Hebrew Bible; they are "doublets" reflecting similar periods of time but containing different content. Samuel (influenced according to this writing under the direction of King David) lists all the gory detail and personal missteps of David's march to kingship and the City of David. However, the book of Samuel makes no reference to David's "blood on hands." That task was accomplished – perhaps under the influence of King Solomon - in the book called Chronicles. After listing David's various victories on the way to the united Israel, the Chronicles clearly state the reason that David could not build the temple: too much blood on his hands. Are you surprised that Chronicles - if influenced by Solomon - never mentioned Bathsheba?

Perhaps, I should complete my letter with a comment of the influence of Parkinson's disease on world history. King David's infirmity gave him early biologic signals of the finality of life which was followed by his intense *focus on purpose*; that focus left him (and us) his gratifying legacy. The combination of severe motor disability and early mortality also was present in the prominent leaders of the Italian Renaissance, the Medici family. Other world leaders stricken with Parkinson's have left a more inglorious path; these include Adolf Hitler and Chairman Mao Tse-Tung. A current dominant world leader remains undiagnosed but has a markedly decreased arm swing; do you know him? (Think Moscow).

Zadok

צדוק

PS: Note to my Christian family

The above dialogue outlines some of the surprisingly shameful aspects of the life of King David - a Biblical hero from our childhood days. At this point, you may wonder why the first verse of the New Testament begins with a reference to David: *"a record of the genealogy of Jesus Christ the son of David."* And then Luke in the book of Acts repeats that God declared *"I have found David son of Jesse a man after my own heart."* Like all mortals, David's life included some shameful events but he never lost Faith or dependency on Yahweh. Scripture from St. Paul also provides clarity: *"It was by faith that David overthrew kingdoms, shut the mouths of lions, and escaped the edge of the sword. His weakness was turned to strength. He earned a good reputation because of his faith, yet he did not receive all that God had promised."* That promise – the promise of the Christian Messiah, the Risen Savior – was foretold in the Davidic covenant and numerous Old Testament passages including the 22nd Psalm.

Behold, the King of Kings!

ABOUT THE AUTHOR

Confession: I never had it in my plans to write a book about Parkinson's disease or King David. At this point in the book, you know that I was blessed with an active surgical career for over three decades. Perhaps my academic publications during the transition from "open" to laparoscopic surgery facilitated my current writing. Also, a high level of introspection during my career transition (read that internal conflict) provided me the background to offer you with this message... which actually was borrowed from King David.

By background, I do not present myself as an expert in Middle Eastern history or biblical studies. As you know by now, I literally stumbled – or should I say *shuffled* - onto the story of David versus Ishbi-Benob. After discovering Ishbi-Benob, I pursued a fairly intense study of the Bible and numerous scholarly works and commentaries. I was surprised that most scholarly commentators gave little or no attention to the battle which, now seemingly, has been so essential to the inspiration and collection of the Psalms as well as Proverbs and Ecclesiastes... and perhaps, even Song of Solomon. At the same time, I was amused that so many so-called scholarly experts have made their mark recently by trying to disprove the authenticity of biblical history rather than to seek its message.

The background materials for this book are available to all. I spent countless hours on the web with YouTube, Wikipedia, and many sources. My biblical references included various translations of the Christian Bible; I found tjjjjhe New Living Translation to read like a novel particularly when dealing with the David story. Also I used the Jewish Scripture called the Tanakh which –for practical purposes - is the same as the Christian Old Testament.

I was surprised at how few influential texts made little to no mention of Ishbi-Benob. These included Charles Swindoll's *David, A Man of Passion and Destiny*; A.W. Pink's *The Life of David*; Jonathan Kirsch's *King David, The Life of the Man Who Ruled Israel;* Baruch Halpern's *David' Secret Demons: Messiah, Murderer, Traitor, King;* Joel Baden's *The Historical David: The Real Life of an Invented Hero;* Israel Finkelstein and Neil Asher Silberman's *David and Solomon*. Robert Alter's *The David Story* mentions Ishbi-Benob in a cursory fashion but it does identify the fragmentary episode as a turning point in David's career. A similar conclusion regarding a career change is made by Robert Barron in his theological commentary entitled *2 Samuel*. After my manuscript was completed, I read several historical fictional accounts. These included Cliff Graham's, Uvi Poznansky, and Elsa Quinones.

Pictured below is a very special lady with her appreciative spouse who happens to be me. She has been my loving wife for nearly 45 years, the mother of my sons and chief literary critic most recently. The photo was taken with an iPhone in an undisclosed location in the Western civilization. Can you recognize it? If not, the answer will be in the next writing. (The mystery location in our first book was Lake Titicaca.)

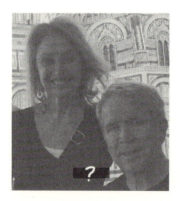

BTW, my first creative writing provides a clue to the location. The short book was entitled *Midnight in Florence: Splattered by Inferno, Sprinkled by Faulkner*. It is all true (mostly) and it is available from Amazon. Why a book about Florence? Not dissimilar to the change in King David's career, the Medici had a familial degenerative arthritis that signaled early mortality preceded by a total loss of mobility.

PARKINSON'S FIRST HERO: KING DAVID

The next writing out of the hopper is intended to be *Parkinson's First Son: King Solomon*. Another writing in the works is *Parkinson's Worst Villain: Adolf Hitler*.

All proceeds from this literary effort will be sent to a special fund for retired surgeons with Parkinson's disease.

"He restoreth my Parkinsonian soul."

Made in the USA
Coppell, TX
20 October 2022